KETOGENIC MEAL PLAN:

The ultimate Beginner's Guide to a detailed and balanced Ketogenic Diet.

I0424340

By Philip Koch.

TABLE OF CONTENTS.

WHY YOU SHOULD READ THIS BOOK.

If you are reading this, it means you want to get into "keto" diet and you've already purchased this book. This book purposely contains detailed information on ketogenic diet for people of all kind. Whatever the condition you have even if prescribed by your doctor, we've got you covered. Make sure to follow the guidelines in this book for the final attainment of the desired results.

INTRODUCTION.

A ketogenic diet refers to a low-carb diet with high fat content which permits the body to produce small energy molecules, the ketones.

Most often, ketogenic diet is a short term diet that is mainly focused on weight loss as it burns down fat more effectively and it also has several benefits to the body including health improvement and overall body performance.

Ketogenic diet is today's most recommended diet by most doctors and is approved for frequent consumption worldwide. This diet's contents are mainly to allow the body systems to get more calories from proteins and fats and equally far much less from carbohydrates.

Carbs that are easily digestible, like sugars, are very much reduced due to the elevated uptake of protein molecules which will in turn be used as a source of energy.

Decreased consumption/intake of carbs by half or its equivalent and consistent amount, the body will sooner or later run out of energy which is mainly the blood sugars that normally provide the a quick access to fuel for immune functions. These processes lead the body to start breaking down the proteins and accumulated fats to act as a source of energy to the body systems through a process known as ketosis.

These actions take place in a very short period of time as it is an alternative energy source to the body when the blood sugar is in short supply. They have an advantage to the body as it helps in the reduction of weight and allow people to achieve some medical conditions like epilepsy, heart and brain diseases, and most importantly acne.

People with some other health conditions like diabetes should therefore consult their doctors first before trying keto in order to get some clear instructions on the best diet associated with their health. Ketogenic diet best suits any kind of health condition whatsoever.

Starvation or better still, fasting, is actually the fastest way to get to the body to produce ketones and get into the metabolic state of ketosis but this is more dangerous as it sounds, because who can really fast for that long time?

With acne, carbohydrates have been mostly associated with this skin condition, so reducing the amount consumed may help in controlling it.

Consumption of a ketogenic diet will lead to the drop in insulin which will eventually stop acne and result in the metabolic process of ketosis which causes weight loss without making yourself starve.

The body breaks down fats on a continuous basis since the body is now accessing energy from the process of fat burning which increases radically as insulin levels decreases.

 The fat stores are now accessible for the break down which is generally countless if one is in the verge of weight loss. This also helps in providing the body systems with a steady supply of energy for metabolism.

This process is made possible through the use of a ketogenic diet.

There still exist some debates and controversies about this kind of diet as to who should be eligible to consume it.

WHO SHOULD AND SHOULD NOT BE ON THIS KIND OF DIET?

There are, however, three groups of individuals that require some special considerations

Are you taking medication for diabetes, like insulin doses?

Are you on high blood pressure/hypertension medications?

Do you breastfeed?

KETO WITH DIABETES.

Whether you have diabetes and still want to try keto, you don't have to panic because this may be the best thing you could ever do to your health for the greater good.

Upon starting low-carb you will need to lower the insulin doses and other doses associated with diabetes have to be reduced a lot.

Ketogenic diet may inverse the type 2 diabetes and bring the blood sugar under control if one happens to have a type 1 diabetes.

The best way of reducing the need to lower the medication is actually through the avoidance of the consumption of carbohydrates that tend to raise the blood sugar level. Insulin doses taken before the adoption of new low-carb keto diet might trigger low blood sugar levels, thus, endangering one's health condition and may result to death.

Therefore your blood sugar needs to occasionally be tested when you are on keto diet and the medication has to be modified accordingly by the doctors best at handling diabetes.

USE OF INSULIN INTYPE 1 DIABETES.

Keto diet with a low-carb and definitely having a high fat content is much effective for consumption by people with type 1 diabetes in order for them to have steady blood sugars.

In the event of frequent hypoglycemia (hypo), a situation where blood sugar level is low, insulin intake should be reduced by dosage before reducing the carb diet intake.

The easiest way to manage a low carb diet is by ensuring the ratio of carbohydrate intake to insulin taken remains the same. This is achieved by less insulin injected into the body as less carbohydrates are consumed.

In some cases of the impacts brought about by protein increasing the quantity of insulin required, then a higher carbohydrate ratio is required.

Other cases where individuals lose weight and increase the sensitivity to insulin under low carb diet, then the ratio of insulin to carbohydrates should automatically be reduced including other insulin doses used.

People with type 1 diabetes occasionally need to use insulin even if they are consuming a very low carbohydrate diet.

A diet having lower than the average amount of carbs each day can eventually lead to ketosis but a strictly low carb diet that has a reasonable protein limitation can lead to a higher and physiological ketone levels.

Insufficient insulin, dehydration and high blood sugar levels can lead to too much production of ketones leading to the occurrence of acidosis, a dangerous complication associated with type 1 diabetes.

When beginning a low-carb diet it is recommended that people with type 1 diabetes should start with an above average quantity of low carb diet per day. At any need for the reduction of the intake amount, a high protein intake should be considered to ensure that there is no development of ketosis.

Starting a low carb diet needs a lot of certainty in order to fully handle the risks but remember that a low carb diet can have pleasing results for people with type 1 diabetes.

INSULIN TREATED TYPE 2 DIABETES.

There is a much likelihood that you will have to stop mealtime insulin if you need to keep on low carb diet. If your blood sugar remains stable continuously, long acting insulin can therefore be able to be reduced.

If at all one takes tablets for diabetes, they should not at all be changed until insulin have been reduced as much as possible. There are instances when some people have the capability of coming out of insulin pretty much completely.

Blood sugar needs to be tested regularly and insulin doses lowered based on the test results. This is so because there is no definitive way of knowing the quantity of insulin that is actually required in advance. A qualified doctor can be of great assistance on this.

Generally, insulin dosses need to be reduced when starting an exacting low carb diet; this is the rule of thumb.

In the event where blood sugar goes a bit high, insulin can be taken later in order to bring it down. Glucose or any other rapid acting carbohydrates can be taken quickly to elevate the blood sugar to a safe level. This clearly reduces the potential influence of low carb diet.

If too much insulin is taken and one ends up having low sugar, it raises concerns since its more dangerous.

INSULIN RELEASING PILLS.

Some pills for type 2 diabetes can bring about low blood sugar level on when one is on a low carb diet. These doses act as stimulators for the pancreas so as to produce more insulin

Sulfonylureas or meglitinides are the major groups upon which pancreas stimulating pills are categorized.

These drugs need to be stopped or the dose be decreased significantly when starting a low carb diet because this will definitely help to avoid lower blood sugar level.

It is recommended that you seek advice from your doctor before getting into it.

KETO DIET WITH HIGH BLOOD PRESSURE.

1. BLOOD-PRESSURE MEDICATION

There is a great risk of actually getting low blood pressure by starting a low carb diet when on blood pressure medication.

It may take several months or a year for this blood pressure dropping effect on a low carb diet to take the full effect if not days.

Dizziness, the feeling getting weak or tiredness is the critical signs that call for blood pressure checkup. If it is low, one has to get in touch with the doctor to stop or reduce the medication.

2. SALT AND BOUILLON

During the first two weeks on a low carb diet, extra fluids and salt should be used in form of bouillon in order to reduce the early side effects that can be worrying mostly during the first week, for example headaches.

This bouillon should only be taken if blood pressure is under control since it can slightly raise the blood pressure.

Extra bouillon or salt should not be taken if the blood pressure remains high even under medication because contrary to that, blood pressure may be raised even higher, which is too risky.

As your body shifts from using glucose to fats as its main source of energy, any form of side effects will appear within some few days.

Keto when Breastfeeding.

Strict Low Carb and Breastfeeding

The body can handle the few carbs that people need to eat under normal conditions. On the other hand, approximately 30 grams or more of sugar is lost per day via milk from breastfeeding.

It is only in rare cases does ketoacidosis occur in the event of not eating carbohydrates while breastfeeding.

Other things like fasting while breastfeeding or having a hard time eating any diet due to sickness can also cause the same situation, not really just the low carb dieting.

It is very important to get enough nutrients while breastfeeding.

How to Eat Low Carb if Breastfeeding

Strict low carb diet should not be eaten if one is breastfeeding, just add some more carbs to be on a safer side since, it will still be effective enough.

At least 50 grams a day is recommended while breastfeeding.

Selecting modest and libera, or enhancing three large fruits per day to an extremely low carb menu is among the ways of getting extra carbs.

KETOGENIC DIET FOODS.

The following list refers to the types of foods that can equally form the low carb menu.

Meat

Fish

Eggs

Vegetables

Natural fats like butter or olive oil.

It is important to stick to foods with fewer than 5% carbs if you are a beginner on this diet.

What to drink.

Drinks like water, coffee, tea or the occasional glass of wine are recommended in this category.

Avoid

Foods which are full of sugar and starch should not be included on a keto diet since they are much higher in carbs.

This is what you should eat on keto.

Meat.

Meats are healthier, low carb and keto friendly especially organic ones.

Note:

Excess proteins are converted to glucose for storage thus making it hard to get into the process of ketosis. Keto is a high fat diet and not protein, therefore, large quantities of meat are not needed.

Processed meats; sausages, meat balls and cold nuts usually contain additional carbs.

Sea foods and fish.

Wild caught fish and salmon is probably the best while breeding should be avoided as it contains carbs.

Eggs.

Organic or pastured eggs can actually be the best and healthiest option, but for other forms of cooked eggs; whether boiled, scrambles or fried, eat then anyway.

Feel free to eat as many eggs as you can but it best not to exceed 35 per day. This is mainly due to the idea of cholesterol.

Natural fat

It is advisable to use fats like coconut fat, olive oil or butter in cooking. High fat sources like garlic butter can delightfully be eaten. Natural sources like eggs, fish, meat are a source of much fats.

SOME OF THE REASONS WHY FATS ARE FINE TO EAT.

Over the years, many science critics have concluded that there is no absolute connection between the saturated fats and heart diseases, which has actually been a mistake.

Fortunate enough, natural saturated fats appear to be neutral from mainly from the health standpoint despite their past research status. This is so due to the fact that more experts and scientific organizations have recently discovered that.

Breast milk and other forms of foods that sustained our ancestors were totally natural, and there is no reason not to eat natural fats which are found in natural foods.

Vegetables growing above the ground.

It is wise to choose vegetables growing above the ground, either frozen or fresh.

These include: cabbage, cauliflower, broccoli, zucchini and avocado.

Vegetables, being boundless and desirable sources of good fat on keto, they can also add color, flavor and some more variety to the keto meal. They can always be fried on butter and add plenty of olive oil into the salad.

Most people starting keto always end up eating much vegetable that before since they start replacing sugary foods.

High-fat dairy.

Butter, cheese and high fat yogurts are good and its advisable to be used in moderation.

Milk can be used sparingly in coffee or tea, but its safe to avoid drinking is in order to avoid adding up the milk sugar levels. Heavy cream can be used for cooking.

The only thing that can slow weight loss is the frequent snacking on cheese when not hungry.

Nuts.

A lot of care has to be taken when using nuts, do not eat more than you need.

Cashew nuts are relatively high carb, better choice is pecan nuts or macadamia as a substitute.

Berries.

A standard amount is good on keto.

Vegetables on Keto

Vegetables basically contain carbs and when the goal is to consume at most 20 grams of per day, veggies with lower carbs are a good option.

Tomatoes being fruits can also be taken on a keto diet but precautions need to be taken since their carbs are a bit higher.

Top 10 Keto Vegetables

The following are the ten peculiar ketogenic vegetables comprising few carbs but with sufficient nutrients.

They are ranked in the order of popularity and the use in ketogenic diet preparation.

Cauliflower.

It is very versatile and has a mild flavor. Used mainly as a base staple like cauliflower mash and rice.

Avocado.

It is full of nutrients and healthy fats event though it is technically a fruit.

Cabbage.

Its tasty when cooked with butter or in stir fry when used as the base.

Broccoli.

Can be steamed, drizzled in cheese, roasted with bacon, and fried in butter and many other ways that makes it tasty and delicious leaving you begging for more.

Spinach.

Can be used in raw salads, creamed or baked into chips since it is a keto friendly low carb vegetable.

Zucchini.

This can be spiralized in order to make a keto pasta.

Asparagus.

It's a great keto vegetable as its very nutritious and low carb

Kale.

Since it has a higher carb, use kale in salads or can be baked into chips.

Green beans.

Can be stewed or cooked in butter or bacon. Other options such as roasting or steaming can still be considered.

Brussels sprouts.

Are tasty when roasted until crispy or can be served in a creamy Sause

Sugar.

Cut all kinds of soft drinks and the sugar water like vitamin water. Also as much as possible, avoid all sugary baking, artificial sweeteners and breakfast cereals.

Starch.

All kinds of potatoes, French fries, rice, bread, potato chips, should be avoided.

Beans and lentils are the legumes with high carbs.

Beer.

There are actually limited low carb beers. Liquid bread containing rapidly absorbed carbs can be a good choice.

Fruit.

Sweet fruits with lots of sugar can only be eaten once in a while.

Also avoid margarine as much as possible since it has no health benefits and it might be linked to asthma, inflammatory diseases and allergies. This is because it has a high content of omega 6.

How much fat do you need to eat?

Carbs and fats are the two main sources of energy to the body. Taking away most carbs means the body will switch to break down fats for energy.

Fats are mainly obtained from the body's fat storage systems or fatty foods.

Keto is popularly called Low Fat High Carb, reason being that it involves eating low carb diet making the body access energy from burning fats, meaning more fats are eaten in the long run.

Fats can be eaten as much as one feels to be contented. A standard quantity of fat has to be maintained because too much of it slows down weight loss and less of it makes you hungry and tired.

Just eat fat when you are hungry and when contented, stop it.

COMMON SIDE EFFECTS ON A KETO DIET

Normally, when people start keto, they experience some side effects mainly relating to dehydration or the lack of the most vital micro nutrients in the body system.

Make sure to stay hydrated and eat consume foods containing high content of micronutrients.

CONSTIPATION

Dehydration is actually the most common cause for constipation and the most probable solution is to increase the water intake as much as a gallon per day.

Fiber content In non-starchy vegetable can also help solve this problem.

A probiotic or husk powder can be helpful if the above doesn't work.

CRAMPS

When beginning ketogenic diet, leg cramps are the most common effects. They occur during the mornings and nights.

Lack of minerals like magnesium in the body is the main cause of these effects.

Taking plenty of fluids and eating salt in the food can help reduce the loss of the mineral, magnesium, and control the issue.

Magnesium supplements can be used only if the problem persists.

HEART PALPITATIONS

On keto transitions, often causes heart to beat faster and more hard. This being a normal condition when doing keto but can still be controlled by taking a lot of water and eating enough salt.

Potassium supplements can be taken at least once a day if the issue persists.

Reduced Physical Performance

Your strength points and stamina may be disturbed a little bit mainly due to the fact that the body shifts towards using fats as a source of energy.

Restrictions can be evident on the normal routines upon beginning ketogenic diet.

Benefits of keto diet can be greatly manifested after working out.

Some of the Less Common Side Effects on a Keto Diet

Most of these problems are related to insufficient micro nutrients and dehydration.

Therefore, it is important to take a lot of water and replenish the electrolytes.

Hair Loss

Multivitamins can be taken if within the first 4 months on keto but it is just a temporary situation.

Though uncommon, hair loss on keto can be put under control by getting enough sleep and making sure that right quantities of calories are taken.

Increased Cholesterol

Higher cholesterol usually has an advantage as it lowers the chances of getting heart disease.

The increment of triglyceride commonly among people in the battle of weight loss will eventually diminish as the weight loss gets back to normal.

Its concluded to be a normal thing when cholesterol elevation occurs in case someone is on keto diet.

BREASTFEEDING

Keto diets are significantly healthy to do while breastfeeding. Addition of extra calories and carbs from fruits can really help when breastfeeding.

300-500 calories significantly contains adde3d fats which help with milk production. Its advisable to consult a medical practitioner on this one.

GALLSTONES

There exists many reports of discomforts upon the start of a ketogenic low carb diet and this is a real downside. Studies, based on gallstones and keto, show that most of the people on keto have either cured or improved gallstones short comings.

Even if your gall bladder is removed, you can still start keto. Fats intake should be on a continuous increase so that the body system gets used to it.

INDIGESTION

Ketogenic diet is known to get rid of indigestion and heartburns upon switching unto it but most people are greatly affected when they are starting out.

The best remedy is to actually reduce the amounts of fat intake as you gradually increase the amounts taken per day for a period of a month.

KETO RASH

Some people happen to itch upon starting keto diet even though there has not been any scientific conclusion to explain it. There is a likelihood that bit be the acetone which excreted through sweat and its also the reason for a bad breath experience.

Taking shower after an exercise is worth looking into.

BONUS ADVICE.

Transition into a ketogenic diet is a little bit hard and toughening but due to the hype about creating a clean and healthy environment for eating makes it easier to find low carb foods. It is usually harder to quantify keto diet in the beginning.

In general, keto diet can have some huge effects on your health for example, changes in body weight, the rise in body energy and mood levels, effect on blood sugar and decrease in body cholesterol

For the first month in keto, keep your carbs low as possible. Be strict on this and always be straightforward about it.

Stay hydrated and keep on supplementing electrolytes since most problems are associated with the lack of electrolytes and frequent dehydration.

Take multivitamins and salt your food but if you still experience the short comings, the advice is to consume electrolyte supplements.

Keep monitoring what you eat in order to avoid overconsuming carbs which are likely to be hidden in everything you eat. This could be helpful in controlling your carb intake rates and make you very much accountable for whatever you let into your body system.

Getting into and maintaining ketosis is significantly dependent on embracing a healthy lifestyle and formulating strategies to cope up with it.

It is of much importance to understand the way your body tends to tolerate stress and by following closely the above stated details, it will be of greater advantage to your body.